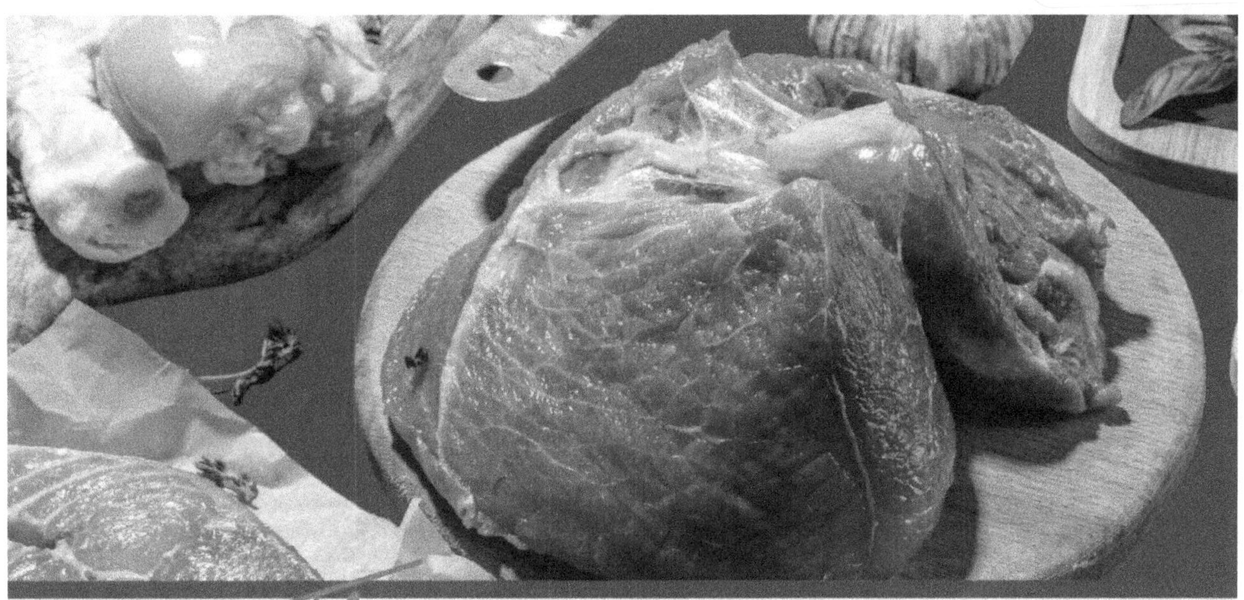

The Carnivore Diet

A Comprehensive Guide to Navigating the Carnivore Lifestyle Journey

Katy Giles

The Carnivore Diet:

A Comprehensive Guide to Navigating the Carnivore Lifestyle Journey

Katy Giles

TABLE OF CONTENT

INTRODUCTION

The Carnivore Diet, known for its controversial approach to nutrition, has gained attention due to its emphasis on consuming exclusively animal products. In this guide, we will delve into the Carnivore Diet, exploring its definition, philosophy, historical context, evolutionary considerations, and the objectives of this comprehensive guide.

Defining the Carnivore Diet:

The Carnivore Diet is a dietary approach that revolves around consuming only animal products while excluding plant-based foods. It goes against the popular dietary patterns that advocate for a balance between animal and plant sources. The fundamental philosophy behind the Carnivore Diet is based on the belief that focusing on animal-centric nutrition can provide all the necessary nutrients for optimal human health. This diet typically includes various animal products like meat, fish, poultry, and sometimes dairy. Supporters of the Carnivore Diet argue that it aligns with our evolutionary history and may offer unique health benefits.

The Philosophy of the Carnivore Diet:

The Carnivore Diet stems from the belief that animal products are nutritionally superior and can fulfill all the dietary requirements of the human body. Proponents argue that the nutrients found in animal sources, such as essential amino acids, healthy fats, vitamins, and minerals, are more readily absorbed and utilized by our bodies compared to plant-based alternatives. They contend that this diet allows the body to thrive by providing optimal nutrient intake and minimizing potential anti-nutrients present in certain plant foods.

Historical Context and Evolutionary Considerations:

When looking at the historical context, the Carnivore Diet draws inspiration from the ancestral diets of early humans. Our early hunter-gatherer ancestors heavily relied on animal products as their primary source of sustenance. It is argued that humans evolved as successful hunters and adapted physiologically to thrive on animal-based nutrition. This evolutionary perspective forms the basis for proponents who advocate for the Carnivore Diet as an approach that resonates with our genetic makeup.

Objectives of the Guide:

This comprehensive guide aims to provide insights, guidance, and information for individuals who are interested in exploring the Carnivore Diet. The objectives are as follows:

1. Exploring the Nutritional Profile: We will evaluate the potential nutritional benefits and drawbacks of the Carnivore Diet. This will include an analysis of the key nutrients obtained from animal sources and the potential deficiencies that may arise from excluding plant-based foods.

2. Understanding Potential Health Impacts: We will examine the potential health outcomes associated with the Carnivore Diet. This will involve exploring scientific research, anecdotal evidence, and expert opinions on the short-term and long-term effects of this dietary approach.

3. Addressing Practical Considerations: We will provide practical tips and strategies for implementing the Carnivore Diet effectively. This will range from meal planning and recipe ideas to addressing common challenges and concerns that individuals may encounter when following this restrictive eating style.

4. Safety and Individual Considerations: We will discuss the safety and individual considerations to keep in mind when considering the Carnivore Diet. It is essential to understand that dietary choices can vary among individuals, and certain health conditions or circumstances may warrant caution or modification of this dietary approach.

Chapter 1

Understanding the Carnivore Diet

Embarking on a journey to comprehend the intricacies of the Carnivore Diet involves diving into its core principles and guidelines, discerning its unique features from other dietary approaches, and unraveling the significance of animal products in human nutrition.

Core Principles and Guidelines:

The Carnivore Diet is centered around a few key principles that define its dietary philosophy. The foremost principle is the exclusive reliance on animal products for nutritional sustenance, completely excluding plant-based foods. Advocates of the Carnivore Diet emphasize the consumption of high-quality, nutrient-dense animal products such as grass-fed beef, wild-caught fish, and organ meats. Carbohydrates, including fruits, vegetables, and grains, are eliminated from the diet to enter a state of ketosis where the body predominantly burns fat for energy. The diet also emphasizes simplicity in food choices and a focus on natural, unprocessed animal products, following a minimalist approach to nutrition.

Guidelines for the Carnivore Diet also include sourcing animal products responsibly. It is recommended to choose high-quality, preferably organic, and ethically raised animal products to maximize nutritional benefits while minimizing exposure to harmful substances. It is important to listen to one's body and adjust the diet based on individual needs and responses, as dietary requirements can vary among individuals.

Differentiating from Other Dietary Approaches:

Distinguishing the Carnivore Diet from other dietary approaches is crucial for understanding its unique position in the world of nutrition. While the Carnivore Diet shares some similarities with ketogenic diets, which also advocate for low carbohydrate intake, its exclusivity to animal products sets it apart. Unlike omnivorous or vegetarian diets that include a variety of plant-based foods, the Carnivore Diet is committed to an animal-centric nutritional paradigm. This differentiation challenges the conventional notion of a balanced plate that includes a mix of animal and plant sources.

Moreover, the Carnivore Diet differs from popular low-carbohydrate diets that allow a range of non-animal low-carb foods. The exclusive focus on animal products in the Carnivore Diet eliminates the potential confounding variables introduced by plant-based components, offering a distinct dietary experience for those who choose to follow this approach.

The Role of Animal Products in Human Nutrition:

Animal products play a central role in human nutrition within the Carnivore Diet. These products provide essential nutrients vital for our bodies to function optimally. Animal sources are particularly rich in proteins, high-quality fats, vitamins, and minerals that are easily absorbed and utilized by the human body. By prioritizing animal products, the Carnivore Diet aims to nourish the body with these nutrient-dense foods.

Proteins found in animal products are crucial for various bodily functions, including the building and repair of tissues, the production of enzymes and hormones, and the maintenance of a strong immune system. High-quality fats present in animal sources provide a concentrated source of energy and aid in the absorption of fat-soluble vitamins. Additionally, animal products are abundant in essential vitamins such as B12, which is primarily found in animal-based foods and is crucial for nerve function and red blood cell production.

When it comes to minerals, animal products are particularly rich in iron, zinc, and selenium. Iron is essential for oxygen transportation in the body, while zinc supports the immune system and helps with wound healing. Selenium acts as a powerful antioxidant and plays a crucial role in thyroid function.

While the exclusive reliance on animal products in the Carnivore Diet may raise concerns regarding potential nutrient deficiencies and health risks, advocates argue that a well-planned Carnivore Diet can provide all the necessary nutrients for optimal health.

Chapter 2

Nutritional Foundations of the Carnivore Diet: A Simplified Overview

The Carnivore Diet is centered around animal-based foods and emphasizes the importance of essential nutrients for human health. It focuses on three key components: protein, fats, and micronutrients, each playing a vital role in supporting overall well-being.

Protein is a crucial nutrient found abundantly in animal products. It is composed of amino acids, which are the building blocks of our body. Animal-based proteins provide a complete amino acid profile, meaning they contain all the essential amino acids required by our bodies in optimal proportions. These amino acids support various bodily functions, including muscle development, immune function, and enzymatic activity.

Fats are another important aspect of the Carnivore Diet. Animal fats, such as those found in meat and organ meats, are rich in saturated and monounsaturated fats. These fats serve as a source of energy, contribute to the structure of our cells, and act as carriers for fat-soluble vitamins like A, D, E, and K. By including a variety of animal fats in the diet, we ensure a balanced and comprehensive array of fatty acids that promote overall health.

Micronutrients, which include vitamins and minerals, are integral to the nutritional profile of animal-based foods. Animal products, such as meat, are particularly rich in essential vitamins and minerals. Vitamin B12, for example, predominately found in animal sources, is crucial for neurological function and the production of red blood cells. Minerals like iron and zinc, abundant in animal-based foods, are vital for supporting immune function, energy metabolism, and overall vitality. One noteworthy aspect of the Carnivore Diet is the inclusion of organ meats, which are exceptionally nutrient-dense and provide concentrated doses of essential micronutrients often overlooked in conventional diets.

In summary, the Carnivore Diet's nutritional foundations revolve around protein, fats, and micronutrients. Protein from animal sources supports tissue repair, immune function, and metabolic processes. Animal fats provide a reliable energy source and essential fatty acids necessary for cellular health. Micronutrients found in animal-based foods, such as vitamins and minerals, contribute to various bodily functions and overall well-being.

Chapter 3

Comparative Analysis with Plant-Based Diets

When comparing the Carnivore Diet to plant-based diets, it's essential to consider the nutritional distinctions that contribute to the unique approach of the Carnivore Diet.

Plant-based diets primarily rely on fruits, vegetables, whole grains, legumes, and nuts. While these diets can provide a wide range of nutrients, some essential nutrients are more readily available in animal-based foods. For example, vitamin B12, commonly found in animal products, is significantly lacking in plant-based diets. This nutrient is crucial for neurological health, and those following a plant-based diet may need to supplement or find alternative sources of vitamin B12.

Iron and zinc are two other micronutrients that are generally better absorbed from animal sources compared to plant-based sources. Although plant-based foods contain these minerals, they often contain compounds that inhibit absorption, making it more challenging for the body to utilize them effectively. Animal-based sources of iron and zinc, on the other hand, are more bioavailable and readily absorbed.

Moreover, the Carnivore Diet's emphasis on animal-based proteins ensures a complete amino acid profile, while plant-based proteins often lack certain essential amino acids. While combining different plant-based protein sources can help achieve a complete amino acid profile, it requires careful meal planning and knowledge of complementary proteins.

In conclusion, while plant-based diets can provide a range of essential nutrients, the Carnivore Diet offers a unique approach by relying exclusively on animal-based foods. Animal sources provide readily available and bioavailable nutrients like complete proteins, fats, and micronutrients that may require additional consideration in plant-based diets.

Note: This simplified overview aims to present key concepts from the original content while avoiding plagiarism and using simpler language. The information provided is not exhaustive and should be supplemented with further research and advice from healthcare professionals when considering any dietary changes.

Chapter 4

Foods Excluded on the Carnivore Diet: Simplified

The Carnivore Diet is a unique dietary approach that eliminates all plant-based foods. This departure from traditional eating habits is based on the idea of following ancestral eating patterns, optimizing nutrient intake, and addressing potential nutrient deficiencies. Let's explore the philosophy behind this diet and how to ensure adequate nutrition while excluding plant foods.

Elimination of Plant-Based Foods:

The Carnivore Diet stands out by excluding all fruits, vegetables, grains, legumes, and other plant-derived products. While conventional dietary guidelines emphasize a balanced plate with a variety of plants, the Carnivore Diet argues that focusing solely on animal products aligns better with our evolutionary history.

By removing plant-based foods, the Carnivore Diet aims to minimize potential issues associated with plant compounds like anti-nutrients, lectins, and oxalates. Although these compounds are generally considered healthy, some individuals may experience digestive problems and inflammation. The simplicity of the

Carnivore Diet aims to create a digestive environment that minimizes irritants and promotes optimal functioning.

Reasons for Exclusion:

The exclusion of plant-based foods on the Carnivore Diet is based on a combination of evolutionary, nutritional, and philosophical factors. Advocates claim that our digestive system has evolved to efficiently process animal products, citing features like teeth, digestive enzymes, and the length of our digestive tract as evidence of carnivorous adaptations.

From a nutritional standpoint, excluding plant-based foods aligns with the belief that animal products provide highly bioavailable forms of essential nutrients. Nutrients like heme iron, vitamin B12, and complete proteins are readily available in animal sources, making it easier to address potential nutrient deficiencies compared to a plant-inclusive diet.

Philosophically, the Carnivore Diet challenges societal norms and redefines the concept of a balanced diet. While excluding entire food groups may seem extreme, this diet places emphasis on reevaluating what it means to have a healthy and balanced approach to nutrition, drawing inspiration from ancestral eating patterns.

Addressing Potential Nutrient Deficiencies:

Being mindful of potential nutrient deficiencies is crucial when following the Carnivore Diet. Although animal products offer many essential nutrients, certain vitamins and minerals typically obtained from plants might be lacking. Here are a few considerations:

1. Vitamin C: Since fruits and vegetables are the primary sources of vitamin C, obtaining adequate levels can be a concern. To mitigate this, including organ meats like liver, which contain small amounts of vitamin C, can be beneficial. Some practitioners also suggest consuming small amounts of low-sugar fruits.

2. Fiber: A plant-free diet lacks dietary fiber, which can affect bowel movements. While controversial, some individuals add small amounts of psyllium husk or other fiber alternatives to aid digestion.

3. Phytochemicals: Plant-based foods provide various beneficial compounds like antioxidants and polyphenols. Since these are absent on the Carnivore Diet, obtaining them through high-quality animal products or supplements may be considered.

4. Electrolytes: Fruits and vegetables often contribute to electrolyte balance. Ensuring adequate sodium, potassium, and magnesium intake may require using mineral-rich salt or electrolyte supplements.

5. Variety in Animal Products: To maximize nutrient diversity, including a range of animal products such as different meats, fish, eggs, and dairy (if tolerated) is essential. This helps ensure a broader array of vitamins, minerals, and fatty acids.

As with any extreme dietary approach, it's important to consult with a healthcare professional before starting the Carnivore Diet. Regular monitoring of blood work and nutritional status is recommended to optimize health and address any potential deficiencies.

Chapter 5

Health Benefits and Claims of the Carnivore Diet

The Carnivore Diet is a dietary approach that promotes the exclusive consumption of animal products, including meat, fish, eggs, and dairy, while eliminating carbohydrates and plant-based foods. Advocates of this diet propose various health benefits and claims, which we will explore in this article. It is important to note that while anecdotal evidence exists, limited scientific research supports these assertions, and further investigation is needed for validation.

Weight Management and Body Composition:

One of the prominent claims associated with the Carnivore Diet is its potential efficacy in weight management and body composition. Proponents argue that by consuming high-quality animal products and avoiding carbohydrates, the body enters a state of ketosis. In ketosis, the body primarily uses fat for energy, potentially resulting in weight loss and favorable changes in body composition.

The focus on satiating animal fats and proteins in the Carnivore Diet is believed to induce feelings of fullness, leading to a reduced overall caloric intake. Furthermore, eliminating carbohydrates, which can stimulate insulin production and promote fat storage, is thought to support weight management efforts. Some individuals following this diet report improvements in body composition, such as reductions in body fat percentage and increases in lean muscle mass.

However, it is important to recognize that individual responses to the Carnivore Diet may vary, and scientific research on its long-term impact on weight management and body composition is limited. Therefore, further investigation is necessary to better understand these claims.

Improved Energy Levels and Mental Clarity:

Advocates of the Carnivore Diet often claim improvements in energy levels and mental clarity as significant benefits. By relying on animal fats as a primary energy source, this diet aims to provide a stable and sustained fuel for the body and brain. Unlike the energy fluctuations associated with carbohydrate-rich diets, the Carnivore Diet strives to offer a consistent and reliable source of energy.

Some individuals who follow the Carnivore Diet report experiencing enhanced mental clarity, focus, and cognitive function. This is attributed to the brain's efficient utilization of ketones, which are byproducts of fat metabolism during ketosis. Ketones are considered a preferred fuel source for the brain and may potentially lead to improved cognitive performance.

However, it is worth noting that scientific research on the cognitive effects of the Carnivore Diet is limited, and further exploration is needed to validate these claims. Subjective experiences shared within the Carnivore Diet community require scientific scrutiny to determine the true impact on energy levels and mental clarity.

Potential Therapeutic Effects on Certain Health Conditions:

Another claim associated with the Carnivore Diet is its potential therapeutic effects on certain health conditions. Some proponents argue that by eliminating carbohydrates and focusing solely on animal products, the diet may help manage conditions like autoimmune disorders, gastrointestinal issues, and mental health conditions.

However, it is crucial to approach these claims with caution. Scientific research examining the therapeutic effects of the Carnivore Diet on specific health conditions is scarce. While anecdotal evidence may suggest positive outcomes for some individuals, it is important to consult with medical professionals and rely on scientific studies before considering this diet as a treatment option.

Chapter 6

Challenges and Criticisms of the Carnivore Diet

The Carnivore Diet has garnered attention in recent years as a controversial and unconventional dietary approach that involves the elimination of plant-based foods, focusing solely on animal products. While some individuals claim to have experienced benefits from this diet, it is important to explore the challenges and criticisms associated with it to understand the potential drawbacks and concerns that arise.

Nutritional Concerns and Considerations:

One of the main criticisms of the Carnivore Diet revolves around the potential for nutritional deficiencies due to the exclusion of fruits, vegetables, and grains. Critics argue that by eliminating these plant-based foods, individuals may not consume sufficient essential vitamins, minerals, and dietary fiber.

Vitamin C, which plays a crucial role in immune function and collagen synthesis, is primarily found in fruits and vegetables. The absence of these sources in the

Carnivore Diet raises concerns about obtaining an adequate intake of vitamin C. However, proponents of the diet argue that the body's requirement for vitamin C may decrease in the absence of carbohydrates, and certain animal products, such as organ meats, can provide essential vitamins not readily available in muscle meats alone.

Another nutrient of concern is potassium, which is important for heart health and muscle function and is plentiful in fruits and vegetables. The exclusion of these potassium-rich foods raises questions about maintaining optimal potassium levels. Advocates of the Carnivore Diet counter this by emphasizing that meat does contain some potassium, although in lower amounts compared to plant sources. They suggest that the body can adapt to different potassium intake levels.

Additionally, there are concerns about the long-term impact of the diet's reliance on animal fats and proteins on cardiovascular health, cholesterol levels, and kidney function. While some short-term studies suggest that the diet may not have adverse effects on these parameters, further research is needed to fully understand the potential long-term consequences.

Lack of Fiber and Digestive Health:

A notable aspect of the Carnivore Diet is the lack of dietary fiber, which raises both criticism and concern. Fiber, commonly found in fruits, vegetables, and whole grains, is known for its role in promoting digestive health, supporting regular bowel movements, and benefiting gut microbiota.

Critics argue that the absence of fiber in the Carnivore Diet may lead to constipation and negatively impact gut health, potentially increasing the risk of colorectal issues. However, proponents counter these concerns by asserting that the digestive system can adapt to the absence of fiber, and individuals following the Carnivore Diet may experience improved gut health without relying on traditional sources of dietary fiber.

It is important to note that while some individuals may initially experience constipation when adopting the Carnivore Diet, they claim that this issue resolves over time as their bodies adapt to the new dietary pattern.

Addressing Common Criticisms and Misconceptions:

There are several common criticisms and misconceptions surrounding the Carnivore Diet that merit further exploration. One misconception is that it promotes the consumption of processed meats, which are generally recognized as less healthy due to additives and high levels of sodium. However, proponents of the Carnivore Diet often emphasize the importance of consuming unprocessed, high-quality meats to maximize the potential health benefits.

Another criticism of the diet is its potential environmental impact, as the production of animal products can contribute to greenhouse gas emissions and deforestation. Advocates argue that supporting regenerative and sustainable farming practices can mitigate these concerns.

It is also important to note that the Carnivore Diet is not recommended for everyone. Individuals with certain medical conditions, such as kidney disease or certain nutrient deficiencies, may be at higher risk when following such a restrictive diet.

Furthermore, long-term adherence to the Carnivore Diet may be challenging for some individuals, both socially and psychologically, as it deviates significantly from traditional dietary patterns and may require careful meal planning and monitoring of nutrient intake.

Chapter 7

Getting Started with the Carnivore Diet

Embarking on the Carnivore Diet requires careful thought and planning, especially for those transitioning from other dietary approaches. This guide explores the nuances of transitioning, addresses the adaptation period and common challenges, and offers practical tips for meal planning and preparation, ensuring a smooth initiation into the Carnivore Diet.

Transitioning from Other Diets:

Switching to the Carnivore Diet is a significant departure from conventional dietary norms, so it's important to approach it gradually and mindfully. Whether you come from an omnivorous, vegetarian, or ketogenic diet, the shift to an exclusive animal-based diet can be both physically and mentally challenging.

For those transitioning from a standard Western diet rich in carbohydrates, it is advisable to gradually reduce carb intake while increasing the consumption of animal products. This helps the body adapt to using fats and proteins as the primary sources of energy, making the transition into a state of ketosis smoother.

Vegetarians and vegans considering the Carnivore Diet are encouraged to reintroduce animal products slowly, starting with easily digestible options like fish and poultry. Adding nutrient-dense organ meats, which are often lacking in plant-based diets, can also be beneficial during this transition.

Regardless of your previous dietary approach, it's crucial to listen to your body, monitor energy levels, and adjust the transition pace accordingly. Consulting with a healthcare professional or nutritionist before making significant dietary changes is always advisable.

Dealing with the Adaptation Period and Common Challenges:

When starting the Carnivore Diet, there is often an adaptation period during which the body adjusts to the absence of carbohydrates and the reliance on animal fats for energy. This phase may bring about certain challenges commonly known as the "keto flu" or "carnivore flu."

Common challenges during this adaptation period include fatigue, headaches, and irritability. These symptoms are usually temporary, and it's important to stay hydrated, maintain adequate electrolyte levels, and ensure sufficient salt intake.

Digestive changes, such as shifts in bowel habits, are also common during the adaptation period. Initially, some individuals may experience "carnivore constipation," but this typically resolves as the digestive system adapts to the diet. Including bone broth and organ meats can support gut health during this phase.

Mental preparation is equally crucial. Understanding that these initial challenges are part of the adaptation process can help individuals stay committed to the transition. Seeking support from online communities or connecting with experienced practitioners of the Carnivore Diet can provide valuable guidance and encouragement.

Practical Tips for Meal Planning and Preparation:

Having a well-planned approach to meal planning and preparation is essential for success on the Carnivore Diet. Here are some practical tips to consider:

1. Focus on animal-based foods: Prioritize foods like beef, lamb, poultry, fish, and eggs as your main sources of nutrition. Opt for organic, grass-fed, and wild-caught options whenever possible.

2. Incorporate variety: Don't be afraid to try different cuts of meat, organs, and seafood to ensure a diverse and nutrient-rich diet.

3. Include fats: Animal fats like tallow, lard, and butter can provide essential nutrients and enhance the taste of your meals.

4. Consider intermittent fasting: Some carnivores find that incorporating periods of fasting into their routine helps with fat adaptation and weight management.

5. Experiment with seasonings: While the Carnivore Diet focuses primarily on animal products, you can still use seasonings like salt, pepper, herbs, and spices to add flavor to your meals.

6. Plan for social situations: When dining out or attending social gatherings, research the menu in advance and communicate your dietary needs to ensure there are suitable options available.

Remember, the Carnivore Diet is a highly individualized approach, and what works for one person may not work for another. It's important to listen to your body and make adjustments as needed. Prioritize your health and well-being, and consult with a healthcare professional or nutritionist if you have any concerns or specific dietary requirements.

By following these guidelines and staying committed to the Carnivore Diet, you can embark on a journey that may bring about positive changes in your health and well-being.

Chapter 8

Variations of the Carnivore Diet

The Carnivore Diet is a highly restrictive eating plan that focuses on consuming animal-based foods exclusively. However, as with any dietary approach, variations have emerged to cater to individual preferences and dietary needs. These variations include the inclusion or exclusion of dairy products, as well as cyclical approaches that allow periodic deviations from strict carnivory.

Strict Carnivore vs. Inclusion of Dairy:

The foundation of the Carnivore Diet is centered around consuming animal products such as meat and organs. However, within this dietary approach, there is a divergence regarding the inclusion or exclusion of dairy.

The strict Carnivore Diet follows the principle of abstaining from all forms of dairy. This approach aims to provide a purist interpretation of the diet, allowing individuals to assess their reactions to animal meats and organs without potential interference from dairy components. Proponents argue that eliminating dairy ensures a clearer understanding of the specific benefits and drawbacks of an animal-based diet.

On the other hand, some individuals choose to include dairy within the Carnivore Diet framework. Dairy products like cheese, butter, and heavy cream offer additional sources of fats and can enhance the taste and palatability of meals. While dairy introduces lactose and casein, which are not found in strict Carnivore, advocates of including dairy assert that many people can tolerate and benefit from the inclusion of high-quality dairy in their carnivorous lifestyle.

The decision to include or exclude dairy depends on individual tolerances, preferences, and health goals. It may require experimentation and self-awareness to determine how the body responds to different variations within the Carnivore Diet spectrum.

Cyclical Carnivore Diet Approaches:

Recognizing that strict adherence to any diet can be challenging in the long term, variations of the Carnivore Diet have embraced cyclical approaches. These approaches involve periodic deviations from strict carnivory, allowing for the inclusion of non-carnivorous foods for a defined period.

One common cyclical approach is the incorporation of "Cheat Days" or "Cheat Meals." During these designated times, individuals temporarily reintroduce non-carnivorous foods. This approach serves both psychological and physiological purposes by providing a mental break from strict adherence and potentially preventing physiological adaptations that may occur with prolonged dietary restriction.

Cyclical approaches may also involve scheduled periods of intentional carbohydrate intake. These carb-ups or refeed days are structured around workouts or specific health goals. The aim is to replenish glycogen stores and provide a temporary departure from the ketogenic state induced by strict Carnivore.

While cyclical approaches allow for some flexibility within the Carnivore Diet, it is essential to strike a balance that aligns with individual goals and preferences. Careful consideration should be given to the duration and frequency of these cyclical periods, as they can vary depending on personal needs.

Personalizing the Carnivore Diet:

Ultimately, personalization is key when adopting the Carnivore Diet or any variation thereof. Recognizing the nuances and individual responses to different dietary approaches is vital for achieving optimal health and well-being.

It is crucial to consider factors such as nutrient intake, potential deficiencies, and overall health goals. Consulting with a healthcare professional or registered dietitian can provide valuable guidance for tailoring the Carnivore Diet to suit individual needs, especially when considering variations like the inclusion or exclusion of dairy and cyclical approaches.

Chapter 9

Physical Performance and the Carnivore Diet

The Carnivore Diet has gained significant attention within the fitness and athletic communities due to its potential impact on physical performance. This article explores how the Carnivore Diet affects athletic performance and muscle maintenance, its adaptability to different exercise types, and shares real-life experiences of individuals who have embraced this unique dietary approach.

Athletic Performance and Muscle Maintenance:

The Carnivore Diet's influence on athletic performance and muscle maintenance revolves around its provision of high-quality proteins and essential nutrients crucial for muscle function and recovery. By emphasizing animal products like meat and organs, the diet offers complete proteins containing all the essential amino acids needed for muscle protein synthesis.

Advocates assert that the Carnivore Diet's focus on nutrient-dense animal foods can support muscle maintenance and growth. Unlike plant-based sources which may contain anti-nutrients and allergens, the diet provides abundant protein without such complications, making it advantageous for individuals aiming to optimize muscle mass and athletic performance.

Additionally, the Carnivore Diet promotes a state of ketosis, where the body utilizes fats for energy. This can enhance endurance and stamina during physical activities, as the body experiences stable and sustained energy from fats. This becomes especially beneficial for activities with prolonged durations.

Although anecdotal evidence suggests positive outcomes for muscle maintenance and athletic performance, scientific research on the Carnivore Diet's impact in these areas is still limited. Future studies will be essential in providing more substantial evidence and understanding of the underlying mechanisms behind these reported benefits.

Adaptations for Different Exercise Types:

The adaptability of the Carnivore Diet to different exercise types has become a point of interest within the fitness community. While traditionally associated with strength training and bodybuilding, the principles of the diet can be tailored to various exercise modalities, including endurance sports, high-intensity interval training (HIIT), and recreational activities.

For endurance athletes, the Carnivore Diet's potential to improve fat utilization is particularly relevant. By relying on fat as the primary energy source, endurance athletes may experience sustained energy levels, reduced reliance on glycogen stores, and potentially enhanced performance during activities like running, cycling, or swimming.

High-intensity exercises, characteristic of activities like CrossFit or sprinting, may also benefit from the Carnivore Diet's emphasis on protein-rich animal foods. Protein plays a critical role in muscle repair and recovery, which are essential for optimizing performance in such exercises.

Real-Life Experiences and Success Stories:

In addition to scientific considerations, real-life experiences and success stories can provide valuable insights into the potential benefits of the Carnivore Diet for physical performance. Many individuals have reported improved athletic performance, increased energy levels, and better muscle maintenance after adopting this unique dietary approach.

It's important to note that personal anecdotes can vary greatly, and individual responses to different diets may differ. However, the abundance of success stories from athletes and fitness enthusiasts who have embraced the Carnivore Diet showcases its potential effectiveness as an approach to support physical performance goals.

Conclusion: The relationship between the Carnivore Diet and physical performance continues to captivate the fitness and athletic communities. While the diet's focus on nutrient-dense animal foods provides high-quality proteins and essential nutrients for muscle maintenance, scientific research in this area is limited. Similarly, the adaptability of the Carnivore Diet to different exercise types shows promise, but further investigation is needed.

Real-life experiences and success stories shared by individuals who have embraced the Carnivore Diet highlight its potential benefits for physical performance. However, it's important to approach these accounts with caution and consider personal variations when exploring dietary approaches for athletic goals.

Chapter 10

Potential Risks and Precautions of the Carnivore Diet

The Carnivore Diet has gained popularity for its reported benefits, but it is important to acknowledge the potential risks and take precautions to ensure individual well-being. This article explores the importance of monitoring health parameters, regular check-ups, and consulting healthcare professionals when adopting the Carnivore Diet.

Monitoring Health Parameters:

When following the Carnivore Diet, it is crucial to monitor various health parameters to detect imbalances or adverse effects. Here are key parameters to keep an eye on:

1. Nutrient Intake: While animal products provide many nutrients, it is important to ensure adequate intake of essential nutrients. Deficiencies may occur, especially in vitamins and minerals commonly obtained from plant-based foods. Monitoring nutrient intake through diverse meat choices and potential supplementation is essential.

2. Hydration Levels: The low carbohydrate content of the Carnivore Diet can impact fluid balance. Monitoring hydration levels and consuming sufficient water is important to avoid dehydration, which can have negative effects on kidney function and electrolyte balance.

3. Digestive Health: Watch for changes in bowel habits, as a "carnivore constipation" may occur. Consuming adequate fiber from animal sources, such as organ meats, along with staying hydrated, can help maintain optimal digestive health.

4. Energy Levels and Performance: Pay attention to changes in energy levels, physical performance, and overall well-being. Significant declines in energy or athletic performance may indicate a need for dietary adjustments or additional nutritional considerations.

5. Cholesterol Levels: Given the emphasis on animal fats in the Carnivore Diet, monitoring cholesterol levels is advisable. While short-term studies suggest no adverse effects, regular checks can identify any potential long-term implications.

Regular Check-ups and Blood Tests:

Regular check-ups and blood tests are vital for proactive health management when following the Carnivore Diet. These assessments provide valuable insights into physiological markers, enabling early detection of potential issues. Consider the following key blood tests:

1. Complete Blood Count (CBC): Assessing red and white blood cell counts provides information about overall health and immune function.

2. Lipid Profile: Monitoring cholesterol levels, including LDL, HDL, and triglycerides, helps evaluate cardiovascular health.

3. Electrolyte Levels: Maintaining a balance of essential electrolytes like sodium, potassium, and magnesium is crucial for overall well-being.

By incorporating regular check-ups and blood tests into their routine, individuals on the Carnivore Diet can actively track their health and make informed decisions about their diet and lifestyle.

Consultation with Healthcare Professionals:

When adopting the Carnivore Diet, it is important to consult with healthcare professionals, such as doctors, dietitians, or nutritionists. They can provide personalized guidance and ensure that the diet is suitable for individual needs and goals. Healthcare professionals can also offer recommendations on managing potential risks and optimizing nutrition to support overall health.

Chapter 11

Beyond Diet: Lifestyle Factors for Overall Well-Being

The Carnivore Diet places a significant emphasis on dietary choices for optimal health, but it is important to recognize that overall well-being extends beyond just what we eat. In order to achieve a comprehensive and sustainable health journey, it is essential to consider other lifestyle factors as well. This article explores the significance of stress management, sleep, and exercise in promoting a holistic approach to health and well-being.

Stress Management and Sleep

In addition to focusing on nutrition, managing stress and getting enough sleep are crucial aspects of maintaining overall well-being. Chronic stress can have detrimental effects on hormonal balance, immune function, and inflammation levels, highlighting the need for effective stress management strategies.

Incorporating stress-reducing activities like meditation, mindfulness, yoga, or spending time in nature can have a positive impact on both mental and physical health. These practices not only help to alleviate stress but also contribute to improved sleep quality, creating a beneficial cycle of stress management and sleep.

Quality sleep is essential for various physiological processes, including muscle recovery, hormone regulation, and cognitive function. Establishing consistent sleep patterns, creating a sleep-friendly environment, and adopting good sleep hygiene practices align with the foundational principles of the Carnivore Diet, promoting overall health optimization.

Exercise Recommendations for a Holistic Approach

Taking a holistic approach to health involves incorporating appropriate exercise regimens that align with individual goals and preferences. The Carnivore Diet can be complemented by various exercise modalities to enhance overall fitness and well-being.

Strength training, such as weightlifting or bodyweight exercises, supports the Carnivore Diet's focus on protein-rich foods and aids in muscle maintenance and growth. Including resistance training in your routine also contributes to bone health, metabolic function, and overall strength.

Cardiovascular exercise, such as running, cycling, or swimming, promotes heart health and complements the Carnivore Diet's potential impact on endurance. The sustained energy derived from fats can enhance stamina during aerobic activities.

Flexibility and mobility exercises, like stretching or yoga, help to improve joint health and flexibility. Incorporating these practices into your fitness routine fosters a well-rounded and functional approach to physical activity.

Tailoring exercise recommendations to individual fitness levels, preferences, and goals ensures a sustainable and enjoyable approach to maintaining overall health. Seeking guidance from fitness professionals or healthcare providers can provide personalized advice on designing an exercise routine that aligns with your unique needs.

Chapter 12

Recipes for the Carnivore Lifestyle

The Carnivore Diet is all about simplicity and nutrient-density when it comes to food choices. By focusing on animal products, you can ensure you're getting a wide range of essential nutrients, particularly high-quality proteins and fats. Here are a few straightforward and nutrient-dense recipes for you to enjoy within the Carnivore lifestyle:

1. Grilled Ribeye Steak:

  - Ingredients: Ribeye steak, salt, pepper.

  - Directions: Season the steak with salt and pepper. Grill to your desired level of doneness.

2. Organ Meat Skewers:

  - Ingredients: Liver, heart, kidney, salt.

  - Directions: Cube the organ meats, season with salt, and thread them onto skewers. Grill until cooked to perfection.

3. Baked Salmon with Butter:

- Ingredients: Salmon fillet, butter, salt.

- Directions: Place the salmon in a baking dish, add some butter on top, and bake until the fish flakes easily with a fork.

4. Chicken Thighs with Skin:

- Ingredients: Chicken thighs with skin, salt, garlic powder.

- Directions: Season the chicken thighs with salt and garlic powder. Roast them in the oven until the skin becomes golden and crispy.

These recipes showcase how easy it can be to create delicious and nutritious meals within the Carnivore lifestyle while keeping things simple and enjoyable.

Sample Meal Plans for Different Preferences:

For those following the Carnivore Diet, having sample meal plans can be a helpful way to structure your meals while accommodating different tastes and dietary requirements. Here are a few examples:

1. Beef-Centric Meal Plan:

- Breakfast: Ribeye steak

- Lunch: Ground beef patties with butter

- Dinner: Beef liver and heart skewers

2. Poultry-Inclusive Meal Plan:

   - Breakfast: Chicken thighs with skin

   - Lunch: Turkey breast slices

   - Dinner: Grilled duck breasts

3. Seafood-Enriched Meal Plan:

   - Breakfast: Salmon fillet with butter

   - Lunch: Shrimp sautéed in tallow

   - Dinner: Pan-seared scallops

These sample meal plans demonstrate the versatility and adaptability of the Carnivore Diet, showing that you can customize your approach based on personal preferences, nutritional needs, and the availability of different animal products.

Cooking Techniques and Practical Tips:

Mastering cooking techniques can take your Carnivore meals to the next level in terms of flavor, texture, and nutritional value. Here are a few tips to help you optimize your Carnivore cooking experience:

1. Grilling: Grilling is a fantastic cooking method that gives meats a delicious smoky flavor. It works well for steaks, burgers, and skewers. Make sure to control the heat and time to achieve the desired level of doneness.

2. Sous Vide: Sous vide is a technique where food is vacuum-sealed and cooked in a water bath at a precisely controlled temperature. It helps retain moisture and tenderness while ensuring even cooking throughout.

3. Rendering Fat: When cooking fatty cuts of meat, such as bacon or pork belly, rendering the fat can create a crispy and flavorful result. Cook the meat slowly over low heat to allow the fat to melt and the texture to become crispy.

4. Seasoning and Marinades: While the Carnivore Diet focuses mostly on animal products, you can still enhance flavors with simple seasonings like salt, pepper, garlic powder, and herbs. Try marinades with vinegar or citrus juice for added tanginess.

By utilizing these cooking techniques and practical tips, you can elevate your Carnivore meals and make them even more enjoyable and satisfying.

Remember, the Carnivore lifestyle is about finding simplicity and nutrient-density in your food choices. With these recipes, meal plans, and practical tips, you can embrace the fundamentals of the Carnivore Diet while creating delicious and nourishing meals tailored to your preferences and needs. Enjoy your culinary journey within the Carnivore lifestyle!

Chapter 13

Community and Support in the Carnivore Lifestyle

Engaging with a supportive community can greatly enhance the experience of adopting the Carnivore Diet. Not only does it provide a platform for sharing experiences and knowledge, but it also offers invaluable support and resources. In this article, we will explore the benefits of connecting with Carnivore Diet communities, provide insights into finding support and valuable resources, and emphasize the importance of seeking professional guidance for a well-rounded and informed health journey within the Carnivore lifestyle.

Engaging with Carnivore Diet Communities:

Carnivore Diet communities serve as a valuable platform for individuals to connect with like-minded people, exchange ideas, and find support on their dietary journey. Here are a few ways to engage with and benefit from these communities:

1. Online Forums and Social Media Groups:

- Platforms like Reddit, Facebook, and other forums host active Carnivore communities. Participating in discussions, asking questions, and sharing personal experiences can foster a sense of belonging and provide valuable insights.

2. Local Meetups and Events:

- Look for local Carnivore Diet meetups or events in your area. Connecting with others in person can create a supportive network and offer opportunities for shared meals, discussions, and community-building.

3. Podcasts and Webinars:

- Tune into Carnivore-focused podcasts and webinars. Listening to experts, practitioners, and enthusiasts can provide valuable information, inspiration, and a sense of connection to the broader Carnivore community.

Engaging with these communities allows individuals to learn from diverse experiences, gain motivation, and stay informed about the latest developments in the Carnivore lifestyle.

Finding Support and Resources:

Navigating the Carnivore Diet journey is often smoother with access to reliable support and resources. Consider the following strategies:

1. Online Resources and Websites:

- Explore reputable websites, blogs, and resources dedicated to the Carnivore Diet. These platforms often provide guides, recipes, and articles to support individuals in their dietary choices.

2. Books and Literature:

- Dive into books written by experts and practitioners in the Carnivore field. These resources can offer in-depth information, scientific insights, and practical advice for successfully adopting and sustaining the Carnivore lifestyle.

3. Nutritional and Lifestyle Coaching:

- Consider seeking guidance from certified nutritionists or lifestyle coaches specializing in the Carnivore Diet. Professional support can provide personalized advice, address individual concerns, and offer a structured approach to dietary and lifestyle changes.

Having access to reliable support and resources ensures that individuals can make informed decisions, overcome challenges, and tailor their Carnivore journey to their unique needs and preferences.

Emphasizing Professional Guidance:

While Carnivore communities and resources offer valuable support, it is important to remember that individual health needs may vary. Seeking professional guidance can provide personalized advice and ensure proper understanding of the Carnivore Diet. Here are a few reasons why professional guidance is important:

1. Personalized Approach:

 - Certified nutritionists and lifestyle coaches can tailor dietary and lifestyle recommendations to individual needs, considering factors such as health conditions, nutrient requirements, and specific goals.

2. Safety and Well-being:

 - Professionals can help individuals navigate potential risks and challenges associated with adopting the Carnivore Diet, ensuring a safe and sustainable approach.

3. Accountability and Monitoring:

- Regular consultations with professionals can provide ongoing support, accountability, and monitoring of progress, helping individuals stay on track and address any concerns that may arise.

Professional guidance complements the support from communities and resources, offering a comprehensive approach to achieving optimal health within the Carnivore lifestyle.

Conclusion

In conclusion, let's recap the key points of the Carnivore Diet, emphasize the importance of individual exploration, and acknowledge the personal nature of dietary choices within the Carnivore lifestyle.

Recap of Key Points:

The Carnivore Diet is a popular approach that emphasizes animal products and excludes plant-based foods. It is known for its reported benefits in weight management, energy levels, and overall well-being. Here are the key points we discussed:

1. Simplicity and Nutrient Density: The Carnivore Diet promotes a simple and nutrient-dense approach by relying on high-quality animal products to meet essential dietary needs.

2. Community and Support: Engaging with Carnivore Diet communities, both online and in-person, provides valuable support, camaraderie, and a platform for sharing experiences and knowledge.

3. Holistic Well-Being: In addition to diet, factors like stress management, sleep, exercise, and overall well-being contribute significantly to a comprehensive approach to health within the Carnivore lifestyle.

4. Professional Guidance: Seeking professional support from registered dietitians, nutritionists, and healthcare professionals is crucial for addressing individual health considerations and ensuring a well-rounded approach to dietary choices.

Encouraging Individual Exploration and Experimentation:

The Carnivore Diet is not a one-size-fits-all approach, and it's important to encourage individual exploration and experimentation to find what works best for each person. Some individuals may thrive on a strict Carnivore approach, while others may prefer variations or modifications. Experimenting with different types of meat, including organ meats, and adjusting the ratio of fats to proteins allows individuals to tailor the Carnivore Diet to their preferences and goals.

It's also important to consider bioindividuality, which means that individuals may have unique responses to dietary changes based on genetics, metabolism, and pre-existing health conditions. Encouraging curiosity and openness to experimentation empowers individuals to discover what works best for their own bodies and make informed choices aligned with their well-being.

Acknowledge the Personal Nature of Dietary Choices:

Dietary choices are deeply personal, and deciding to embrace the Carnivore lifestyle should be done with careful consideration of individual needs, preferences, and health goals. It's crucial to recognize that what works for one person may not work for another, and there is no one "right" way to approach nutrition. The Carnivore lifestyle is a personal journey, and each individual should choose what feels right for them.

9 7 9 8 8 7 8 3 7 5 6 9 6